HEART HEALTHY COOKBOOK FOR BEGINNERS 2024

Delicious and Easy Recipes to Lower Your Blood Pressure, Improve and Reverse Your Heart Disease

DARREN RUIZ

TABLE OF CONTENTS

CHAPTER 9 : VEGETARIAN RECIPES

<u>Sweet Potato and Spinach Salad</u>

<u>Caprese Stuffed Avocado</u>

<u>Tofu and Broccoli Stir-Fry</u>

<u>Mushroom and Spinach Quesadilla</u>

<u>Butternut Squash and Black Bean Chili</u>

CONCLUSION

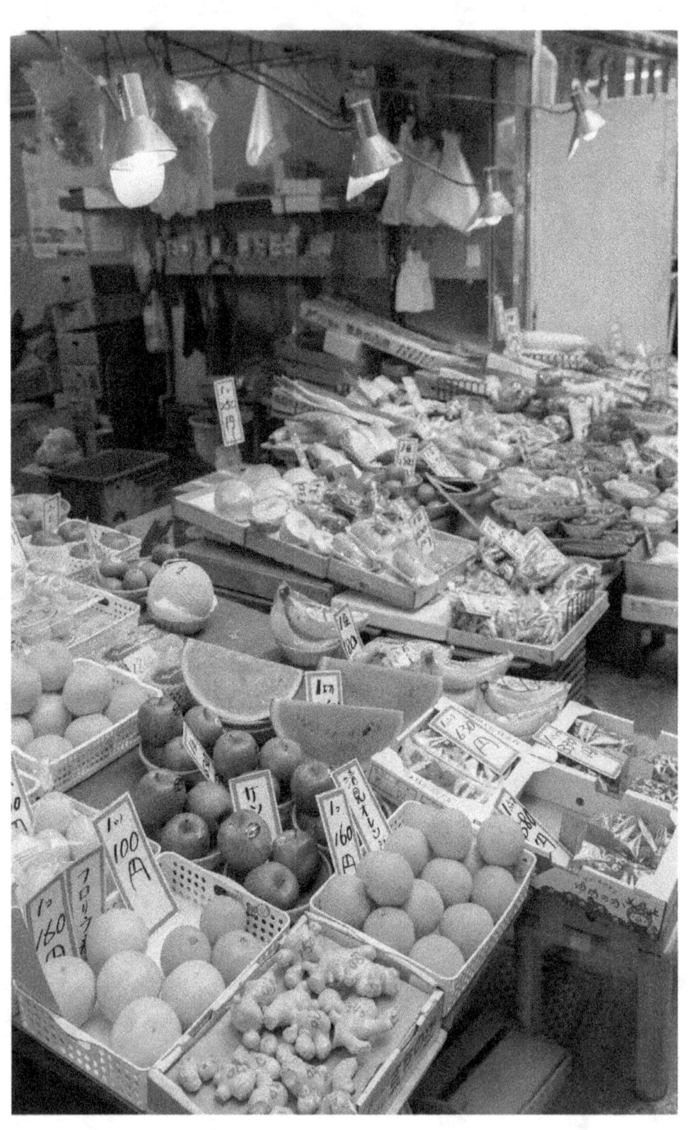

INTRODUCTION

In a quaint, sunlit village nestled among rolling hills, there lived an old man named Samuel. Samuel was a fixture in the community, known for his hearty laugh, warm smile, and the twinkle in his eyes that belied his age.

However, beneath that jovial exterior, Samuel had been struggling with heart disease for years. It had sapped his energy, burdened his daily life, and left him feeling like an old man far beyond his years.

One day, Samuel decided that enough was enough. He couldn't bear the thought of missing out on the simple pleasures of life that he once enjoyed, like taking long walks through the meadows or dancing with his grandchildren. With unwavering determination, he set out on a mission to reverse his heart disease and regain his vitality.

Samuel began his journey by seeking the advice of a local nutritionist who had a reputation for helping people make positive changes in their lives through dietary choices.

The nutritionist introduced Samuel to a heart-healthy diet that emphasised fresh fruits and vegetables, whole grains, lean protein, and unsaturated fats. Samuel was initially overwhelmed by the new foods he needed to incorporate into his diet, but he knew it was a crucial step in his quest for a healthier heart.

With a sense of purpose, Samuel embraced his new dietary regimen. He shunned processed foods and replaced them with vibrant, colourful vegetables and fruits that painted a rainbow on his plate.

He traded his fatty meats for lean poultry and fish. Samuel also started cooking with olive oil and using nuts as snacks instead of chips.

The transition wasn't always easy, but he found that the flavours of fresh, wholesome foods soon won him over.

As the months passed, Samuel's perseverance paid off. His energy levels began to surge, and the pounds he had carried for so long began to melt away. His friends and family noticed the change and cheered him on as he continued his heart-healthy journey.

Samuel's dedication to his new lifestyle led to more than just physical improvements; it brought joy back into his life. He found himself taking long, leisurely walks through the meadows, his heart no longer heavy with the burden of disease. He twirled his grandchildren around the living room, their laughter filling the air as they danced together.

Over time, Samuel's visits to the doctor brought increasingly positive news. His heart health improved, his blood pressure normalised, and his cholesterol levels dropped.

The transformation was nothing short of remarkable, and Samuel had reclaimed his vitality and zest for life.

His story became an inspiration in the village, serving as a testament to the power of making the right dietary choices.

Samuel's journey was a reminder that with determination, the right guidance, and a heart full of hope, it was possible to reverse the grip of heart disease and embrace a vibrant and healthy life, no matter one's age. Samuel's heart, once ailing, had now become a symbol of resilience, renewal, and the incredible potential of the human spirit.

CHAPTER 1

Understanding Heart Disease

The heart, an extraordinary organ, relentlessly pumps life-sustaining blood throughout our bodies. However, it is not invincible. Heart disease, a prevalent and often silent threat, can undermine its vital functions.

In this comprehensive exploration, we delve into the various types of heart disease, their root causes, common symptoms, and the crucial preventive measures that can help maintain heart health.

Keeping in mind the inspiring journey of Samuel, the old man who defied the odds to reverse his heart disease through dietary changes.

Types of Heart Disease:

Heart disease is an umbrella term encompassing various cardiovascular conditions that affect the heart and blood vessels. The most prevalent types include:

Coronary Artery Disease (CAD): CAD, also known as atherosclerosis, is characterised by the narrowing of the coronary arteries due to the accumulation of plaque.

This restricts blood flow, often leading to chest pain or angina, and, in severe cases, heart attacks.

Heart Failure: Heart failure occurs when the heart cannot pump blood effectively, causing fluid buildup in the lungs and other parts of the body.

It is not a sudden stoppage but a gradual weakening of the heart's ability to function.

Arrhythmias: Arrhythmias are irregular heart rhythms. They can manifest as tachycardia (fast heart rate) or bradycardia (slow heart rate) and may lead to fainting, palpitations, or dizziness.

Valvular Heart Disease: Valvular heart disease involves abnormalities in the heart's valves, which can lead to regurgitation, stenosis, or prolapse of the valves. Symptoms vary based on the affected valve and the severity of the condition.

Congenital Heart Defects: These are heart abnormalities present at birth, often requiring surgery or ongoing medical care. The symptoms and complications associated with congenital heart defects differ significantly from person to person.

Root Causes of Heart Disease:

Understanding the causes of heart disease is pivotal in addressing and preventing it. Key contributing factors include:

Atherosclerosis: The buildup of cholesterol-rich plaque in the arteries is a primary cause of coronary artery disease. This restricts blood flow to the heart and can lead to heart attacks.

High Blood Pressure (Hypertension): Elevated blood pressure forces the heart to work harder, potentially leading to heart failure, stroke, or other cardiovascular complications.

Diabetes: Uncontrolled diabetes can damage blood vessels and nerves, increasing the risk of heart disease.

Smoking: Tobacco use damages blood vessels, increases blood pressure, and lowers good cholesterol levels, contributing to heart disease.

High Cholesterol: Elevated levels of low-density lipoprotein (LDL) cholesterol can lead to atherosclerosis and coronary artery disease.

Obesity: Being overweight or obese strains the heart, raises blood pressure, and increases the risk of heart disease.

Sedentary Lifestyle: Lack of physical activity weakens the heart and contributes to obesity, high blood pressure, and diabetes.

Recognizing Symptoms:

Identifying the early signs of heart disease is crucial for timely intervention and treatment. Symptoms may vary depending on the specific condition but often include:

- Chest pain or discomfort (angina) that may radiate to the arms, neck, jaw, or back.
- Shortness of breath, especially during physical activity.
- Fatigue and weakness.
- Rapid or irregular heartbeat (palpitations).

- Swelling in the legs, ankles, or abdomen.
- Dizziness, lightheadedness, or fainting.
- Cold sweats.

Preventive Measures:

Heart disease is not an inevitability; there are steps that can be taken to reduce its risk and manage its effects. Samuel's remarkable journey of reversing heart disease through dietary changes serves as a testament to the effectiveness of preventive measures.

Diet and Nutrition:

A heart-healthy diet can significantly lower the risk of heart disease. Focus on:

- A diet rich in fruits and vegetables to provide essential vitamins, minerals, and antioxidants.

- Whole grains, such as whole wheat, oats, and brown rice, to increase dietary fibre.
- Lean protein sources like poultry, fish, beans, and legumes while reducing red meat consumption.
- Unsaturated fats, including olive oil and avocados, to replace saturated fats and trans fats.
- Limiting salt intake to control blood pressure.
- Reducing sugar and processed food consumption.

Physical Activity:

Regular exercise is vital for heart health. Aim for at least 150 minutes of moderate-intensity aerobic activity or 75 minutes of vigorous-intensity activity per week. Incorporating strength training and flexibility exercises can further enhance heart health.

Smoking Cessation:

Quitting smoking is one of the most impactful steps one can take to improve heart health. It reduces the risk of atherosclerosis and lowers blood pressure.

Weight Management:

Maintaining a healthy weight through a balanced diet and regular exercise helps reduce the strain on the heart.

Managing Chronic Conditions:

For individuals with conditions like diabetes or high blood pressure, diligent management and medication adherence are key to preventing heart disease.

Regular Check-Ups:

Annual check-ups and screenings can detect early signs of heart disease or its risk factors.

Monitoring blood pressure, cholesterol levels, and diabetes is essential.

Stress Management:

Chronic stress can negatively impact heart health. Practising stress-reduction techniques such as mindfulness, meditation, and hobbies can be beneficial.

Heart disease, in all its forms, is a formidable adversary, but it is not insurmountable.

The inspiring story of Samuel underscores the power of positive lifestyle changes, particularly in the realm of diet and nutrition, to reverse the effects of heart disease and embrace a vibrant, healthy life.

Understanding the different types of heart disease, their root causes, recognizing symptoms, and taking preventive measures can significantly reduce the risk of this pervasive condition.

With knowledge, determination, and a commitment to heart-healthy living, we can all take steps to protect and cherish our hearts for years to come.

CHAPTER 2

Nourishing Your Heart

Maintaining a heart-healthy diet is a pivotal step in reducing the risk of heart disease and promoting overall cardiovascular well-being. Understanding the foods to include and those to avoid is essential to achieve optimum health for your heart.

Foods to Embrace:

Fruits and Vegetables:

Colourful fruits and vegetables like berries, citrus fruits, leafy greens, and bell peppers are rich in vitamins, minerals, and antioxidants that support heart health.

Their high fibre content aids in lowering cholesterol levels and reducing the risk of heart disease.

Whole Grains:

Whole grains, such as oats, quinoa, brown rice, and whole wheat, are excellent sources of dietary fibre and essential nutrients.They help regulate blood sugar, lower cholesterol, and maintain healthy blood pressure.

Lean Protein:

Choose lean protein sources like skinless poultry, fish, beans, lentils, and tofu.These options are low in saturated fat and can replace red meat in your diet, reducing the risk of heart disease.

Fatty Fish:

Fatty fish like salmon, mackerel, and trout are rich in omega-3 fatty acids, which are known to reduce the risk of heart disease.Aim to incorporate fish into your diet at least twice a week.

Nuts and Seeds:

Almonds, walnuts, chia seeds, and flaxseeds are packed with heart-healthy nutrients, including fiber, healthy fats, and antioxidants.A handful of nuts or a sprinkle of seeds can be a nutritious snack.

Legumes:

Beans, lentils, and chickpeas are high in fiber, protein, and essential minerals.They can help lower cholesterol and manage blood sugar levels.

Foods to Avoid:

Saturated and Trans Fats:

Limit your intake of saturated fats found in red meat, full-fat dairy products, and processed foods.Trans fats, often found in fried and baked goods, should be avoided altogether as they raise bad cholesterol levels.

Processed Foods:

Highly processed foods, such as sugary snacks, sugary beverages, and fast food, are often laden with unhealthy fats, sugars, and excessive salt.Consuming these foods can contribute to obesity and heart disease.

Excessive Salt:

High sodium intake can lead to elevated blood pressure, increasing the risk of heart disease and stroke.

Limit your consumption of salty processed foods and season your meals with herbs and spices instead.

Refined Grains:

Refined grains like white bread, white rice, and sugary cereals lack the fiber and nutrients found in whole grains.These foods can lead to blood sugar spikes and contribute to heart disease.

Added Sugars:

Sugary foods and beverages can raise triglyceride levels, promoting inflammation and increasing the risk of heart disease.

Be mindful of hidden sugars in processed foods and opt for natural sweeteners like honey or maple syrup in moderation.

Excessive Alcohol:

While moderate alcohol consumption may have heart benefits, excessive drinking can lead to high blood pressure, obesity, and other cardiovascular issues.If you choose to consume alcohol, do so in moderation.

By adopting these dietary guidelines, you can take a significant step towards reducing the risk of heart disease and achieving optimal heart health.

Remember, small changes in your diet can lead to significant improvements in your heart's well-being, allowing you to enjoy a long and healthy life.

Core Benefits of Following A Heart Healthy Disease Diet

Embracing a heart-healthy diet, especially for beginners, offers a range of core benefits that can significantly enhance overall well-being and reduce the risk of heart disease. Here are the key advantages of adopting such a diet:

Cardiovascular Health: A heart-healthy diet helps improve heart health by reducing the risk of heart disease, lowering blood pressure, and managing cholesterol levels.

Weight Management: By focusing on nutritious, whole foods and portion control, a heart-healthy diet assists in achieving and maintaining a healthy weight.

This is essential because obesity is a major risk factor for heart disease.

Blood Pressure Control: A diet rich in fruits, vegetables, and whole grains, and low in sodium, helps regulate blood pressure. Lowering high blood pressure is crucial in preventing heart disease and its complications.

Cholesterol Reduction: Consuming foods with healthy fats, such as those found in nuts, seeds, and fatty fish, can help lower bad cholesterol (LDL) levels and raise good cholesterol (HDL) levels.

Blood Sugar Management: Whole grains, fibre-rich foods, and balanced carbohydrate intake in a heart-healthy diet assist in controlling blood sugar levels.

Inflammation Reduction: Certain foods in a heart-healthy diet, particularly those high in antioxidants and omega-3 fatty acids, have anti-inflammatory properties.

Chronic inflammation is linked to heart disease, and reducing it can improve heart health.

Digestive Health: A diet rich in fibre from fruits, vegetables, and whole grains supports digestive health. This can help prevent digestive issues and maintain overall well-being.

Risk Reduction for Chronic Diseases: Adopting a heart-healthy diet not only reduces the risk of heart disease but also lowers the risk of other chronic conditions like type 2 diabetes, certain cancers, and obesity.

Complications of Heart Healthy Disease

The complications of heart disease can be severe and even life-threatening if the right diet isn't adopted. Here are some of the potential complications that may arise when a heart-healthy diet is not followed:

Heart Attack: Failing to adopt a heart-healthy diet increases the risk of a heart attack. A diet high in saturated fats and cholesterol can lead to the buildup of arterial plaque, increasing the likelihood of a blood clot forming and blocking blood flow to the heart.

Stroke: Uncontrolled high blood pressure, often exacerbated by excessive sodium intake, can lead to strokes.

A stroke occurs when a blood vessel in the brain becomes blocked or bursts, resulting in a lack of oxygen to the brain tissue.

High Blood Pressure: A diet rich in sodium and unhealthy fats can contribute to elevated blood pressure.

Untreated high blood pressure is a significant risk factor for heart disease and can lead to heart failure, stroke, or other cardiovascular issues.

Diabetes: Excessive sugar intake and poor dietary habits can lead to obesity and insulin resistance, increasing the risk of type 2 diabetes. Diabetes, in turn, is a major risk factor for heart disease.

Shortened Lifespan: Failing to adopt a heart-healthy diet can significantly reduce life expectancy. Heart disease remains one of the leading causes of death worldwide, and diet plays a crucial role in preventing it.

In conclusion, following a heart-healthy diet as a beginner is a proactive and rewarding step towards a longer, healthier life. It offers a myriad of benefits that encompass not only heart health but also overall physical and mental well-being.

By making mindful food choices and adopting a heart-healthy eating pattern, beginners can take control of their health and reduce their risk of heart disease and related health issues.

CHAPTER 3

How to Follow a Heart Healthy Disease Diet

Following a heart-healthy diet is a proactive approach to maintaining cardiovascular health and reducing the risk of heart disease. It involves making conscious food choices and adopting a dietary pattern that supports overall well-being. Here's a step-by-step guide on how to follow a heart-healthy diet:

Consult a Healthcare Professional: Before making significant dietary changes, it's advisable to consult with a healthcare professional, such as a doctor or a registered dietitian.

They can provide personalised recommendations based on your health status, age, and specific dietary needs.

Educate Yourself: Familiarise yourself with the principles of a heart-healthy diet. Learn about the types of foods that are beneficial for heart health and those that should be limited or avoided.

Understand Portion Control: Pay attention to portion sizes. Even healthy foods can contribute to weight gain if consumed in excess. Using measuring cups or a food scale can help you better understand appropriate portion sizes.

Focus on Whole, Unprocessed Foods: Whole foods, such as fruits, vegetables, whole grains, lean proteins, and healthy fats, should form the foundation of your diet. These foods are rich in nutrients and low in added sugars, salt, and unhealthy fats.

Choose Healthy Fats: Opt for unsaturated fats found in olive oil, avocados, nuts, and seeds. These fats can help lower bad cholesterol (LDL) levels and reduce inflammation in the body.

Lean Protein Sources: Select lean protein options like skinless poultry, fish, beans, lentils, and tofu. Limit red meat, especially processed and high-fat cuts.

Low-Sodium Choices: Be mindful of your sodium intake by choosing low-sodium products and reducing salt in cooking. High sodium levels can lead to high blood pressure, a risk factor for heart disease.

Monitor Cholesterol Intake: Be aware of cholesterol-rich foods, especially those high in saturated and trans fats. Limit your intake of foods like egg yolks and organ meats.

Moderate Alcohol Consumption: If you consume alcohol, do so in moderation. This typically means up to one drink per day for women and up to two drinks per day for men.

Excessive alcohol consumption can have adverse effects on the heart.

Stay Hydrated: Adequate hydration is essential for overall health. Water is the best choice for staying hydrated, as sugary beverages can contribute to weight gain and heart disease.

Regular Exercise: Complement your heart-healthy diet with regular physical activity. Exercise is a crucial component of cardiovascular health.

Track Your Progress: Monitor your dietary choices and keep a food diary if it helps. Regularly review your diet and make adjustments as needed.

10 Healthy Shopping Lists For A Heart-healthy Disease Diet

When following a heart-healthy diet, it's essential to stock your kitchen with ingredients that promote cardiovascular well-being. Here are 20 healthy shopping ingredients for a heart-healthy diet:

Fruits: Choose a variety of fresh fruits, such as apples, berries, oranges, and bananas. They are rich in vitamins, minerals, and antioxidants.

Vegetables: Stock up on colorful vegetables like leafy greens, broccoli, carrots, and bell peppers. They provide essential nutrients and fiber.

Whole Grains: Opt for whole grains like brown rice, quinoa, whole wheat pasta, and oats. They are high in fiber and help regulate blood sugar.

Legumes: Buy beans, lentils, and chickpeas. They are excellent sources of plant-based protein and fiber.

Nuts: Include almonds, walnuts, and pistachios for healthy fats and protein. A handful of nuts makes for a nutritious snack.

Seeds: Purchase flaxseeds, chia seeds, and sunflower seeds. They are rich in heart-healthy omega-3 fatty acids and fibre.

Lean Proteins: Choose skinless poultry, turkey, and lean cuts of beef or pork. Opt for lean proteins to reduce saturated fat intake.

Low-Fat Dairy: Select low-fat or fat-free dairy products like yogurt, milk, and cheese. These options are lower in saturated fat.

Herbs and Spices: Herbs like basil, oregano, and spices such as turmeric, cayenne pepper, and garlic add flavor without salt.

Low-Sodium Broth: Use low-sodium chicken or vegetable broth for soups and stews. It reduces sodium intake.

Meal Planning For Heart-healthy Disease Diet

Meal planning for a heart-healthy diet is a structured approach to preparing and consuming meals that prioritise foods and ingredients beneficial for cardiovascular health. Meal planning offers several benefits for the proper management of heart disease and overall well-being:

Control Over Nutrient Intake: Meal planning allows you to carefully select and control the nutrients in your diet. You can focus on essential nutrients like fibre, vitamins, minerals, and healthy fats while minimising unhealthy components like saturated fats, sodium, and added sugars.

Blood Sugar Management: Planning meals with complex carbohydrates and fibre can help stabilise blood sugar levels. This is particularly important for individuals with or at risk of developing diabetes, a significant risk factor for heart disease.

Increased Fibre Intake: Planning meals with a focus on high-fibre foods like fruits, vegetables, and whole grains promotes digestive health, regulates cholesterol levels, and supports weight management.

Stress Reduction: Knowing what you'll eat and having the necessary ingredients on hand reduces the stress of last-minute meal decisions. Lowering stress can positively impact heart health.

Variety and Enjoyment: A well-thought-out meal plan ensures variety in your diet, making it more enjoyable and less monotonous. This can contribute to the sustainability of a heart-healthy eating pattern.

Healthier Cooking Techniques: Meal planning often involves healthier cooking techniques such as grilling, baking, or steaming, which can reduce the intake of unhealthy fats and lower the risk of heart disease.

7 Days Sample Heart Disease Meal Plan

Day 1:

- **Breakfast:** Greek yoghourt with mixed berries and a sprinkle of chia seeds.
- **Lunch:** Spinach and mushroom salad with a lemon vinaigrette.
- **Snack:** Sliced cucumber with hummus.
- **Dinner:** Baked salmon with quinoa and steamed broccoli.

Day 2:

- **Breakfast:** Oatmeal topped with sliced banana and a drizzle of honey.
- **Lunch:** Lentil and vegetable stir-fry with brown rice.
- **Snack:** Almonds and dried apricots.
- **Dinner:** Grilled chicken breast with a side of sweet potato and mixed greens.

Day 3:

- **Breakfast:** Whole wheat toast with avocado and a poached egg.
- **Lunch:** Chickpea and vegetable curry with a side of quinoa.
- **Snack:** Sliced bell peppers with guacamole.
- **Dinner:** Caprese stuffed avocado.

Day 4:

- **Breakfast:** Smoothie with spinach, banana, almond milk, and a scoop of protein powder.
- **Lunch:** Quinoa and black bean salad.
- **Snack:** Greek yogurt with honey and walnuts.
- **Dinner:** Tofu and broccoli stir-fry with brown rice.

Day 5:

- **Breakfast:** Chia seed pudding with fresh mango.

- **Lunch:** Mushroom and spinach quesadilla.
- **Snack:** Sliced apple with almond butter.
- **Dinner:** Butternut squash and black bean chili.

Day 6:

- **Breakfast:** Scrambled eggs with diced tomatoes and spinach.
- **Lunch:** Lentil and vegetable soup with whole wheat bread.
- **Snack:** Cottage cheese with pineapple.
- **Dinner:** Eggplant and tomato ratatouille.

Day 7:

- **Breakfast:** Whole grain cereal with low-fat milk and a handful of strawberries.
- **Lunch:** Spinach and mushroom stuffed portobello mushrooms.
- **Snack:** Mixed nuts.

- **Dinner:** Quinoa and vegetable stir-fry with tofu.

Feel free to adapt the meal plan based on your preferences and dietary requirements. Remember to stay hydrated and engage in regular physical activity to complement your heart-healthy diet.

By following these steps and embracing a heart-healthy diet, you can significantly reduce the risk of heart disease, improve overall health, and enjoy a long and fulfilling life. Remember that small, sustainable changes can lead to lasting benefits for your heart and well-being.

CHAPTER 4

Easy Breakfast Recipes

Introducing "Easy Breakfast Recipes for Heart Disease" – a collection of delicious and nourishing morning meals designed to support your cardiovascular health.

In this cookbook, you'll discover a variety of breakfast options that are not only satisfying and flavorful but also tailored to reduce your risk of heart disease.

Start your day right and embark on a journey to better heart health with our easy breakfast recipes.

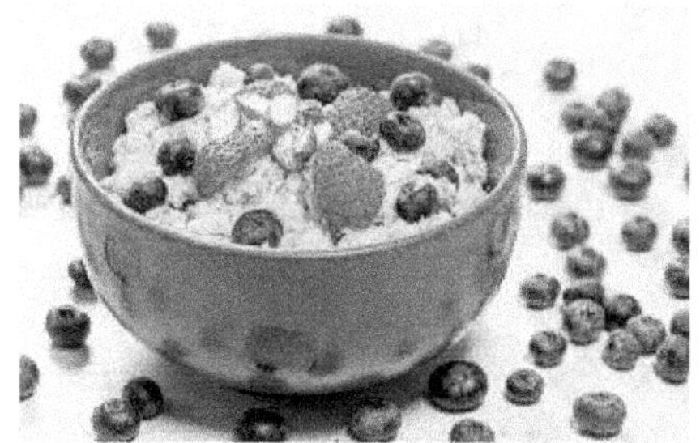

Oatmeal with Berries and Almonds

Ingredients:
- Half cup rolled oats
- One cup water or milk
- One quarter cup berries
- One tablespoon almonds, chopped

Preparation:
- Combine the oats, water or milk, and salt in a saucepan over medium heat.
- Bring to a boil, then reduce heat to low and simmer for 5–7 minutes, or until the oats are cooked through.
- Stir in the berries and almonds and cook for another minute.
- Serve immediately.

Nutritional value: (per serving)
- Calories: 250
- Fat: 5g
- Protein: 10g
- Carbohydrates: 40g
- Fibre: 5g
- Sugar: 5g
- Cooking time: 10–12 minutes

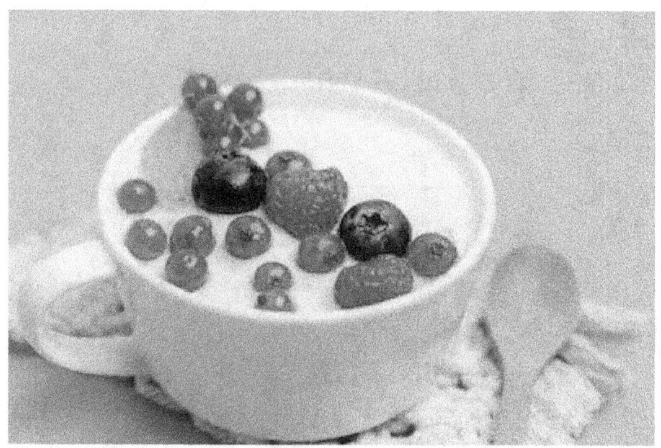

Greek Yoghurt Parfait

Ingredients:
- One cup Greek yogurt
- Half cup berries
- One quarter cup granola

Preparation:
- Layer the Greek yoghurt, berries, and granola in a jar or glass.
- Serve immediately.

Nutritional value: (per serving)
- Calories: 200
- Fat: 5g
- Protein: 15g
- Carbohydrates: 20g
- Fibre: 5g

- Sugar: 10g
- Cooking time: 5 minutes

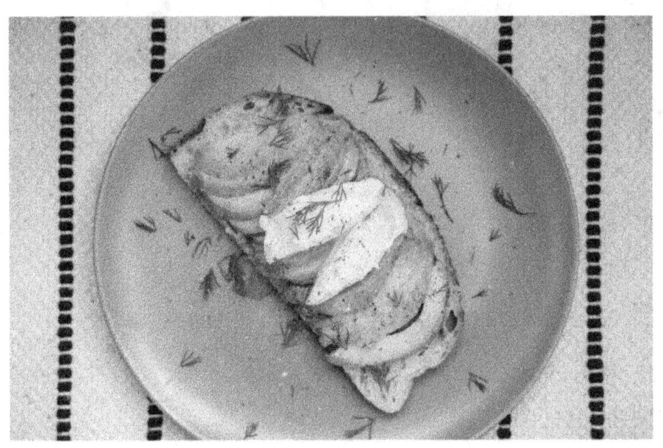

Avocado Toast with Poached Egg

Ingredients:
- One slice whole-grain bread
- One quarter avocado, mashed
- One poached egg
- Salt and pepper to taste

Preparation:
- Toast the bread.
- Spread the mashed avocado on the toast.
- Top with the poached egg and season with salt and pepper to taste.

- Serve immediately.

Nutritional value: (per serving)
- Calories: 250
- Fat: 15g
- Protein: 10g
- Carbohydrates: 20g
- Fiber: 5g
- Sugar: 5g
- Cooking time: 10-12 minutes (including poaching the egg)

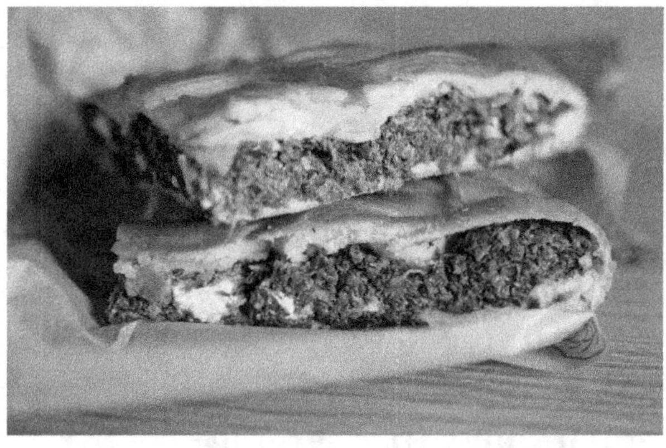

Spinach and Feta Omelette

Ingredients:
- Two eggs
- One quarter cup milk
- One quarter cup spinach, chopped

- One quarter cup feta cheese, crumbled
- Salt and pepper to taste

Preparation:
- Whisk together the eggs, milk, salt, and pepper in a bowl.
- Heat a small non-stick skillet over medium heat.
- Spray the skillet with cooking spray.
- Pour the egg mixture into the skillet.
- When the eggs are set on the bottom, sprinkle with the spinach and feta cheese.
- Fold the omelette in half and cook for another minute, or until the eggs are cooked through.
- Serve immediately.

Nutritional value: (per serving)
- Calories: 200
- Fat: 10g
- Protein: 15g
- Carbohydrates: 5g
- Fiber: 2g
- Sugar: 2g

- Cooking time: 5-7 minutes

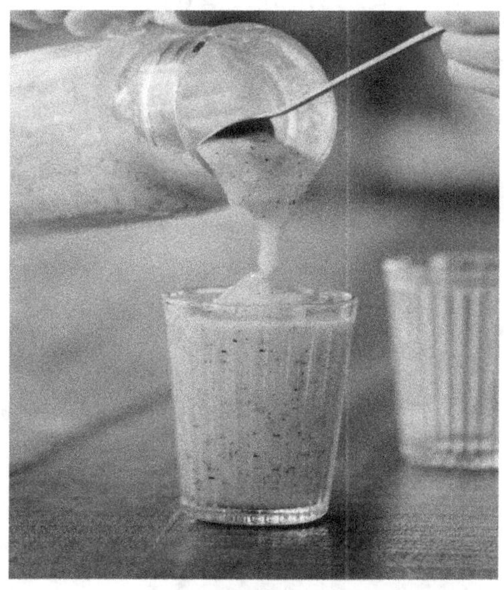

Peanut Butter and Banana Smoothie

Ingredients:
- One cup milk
- Half cup banana, sliced
- One quarter cup peanut butter
- One tablespoon honey (optional)

Preparation:
- Combine all of the ingredients in a blender and blend until smooth.

- Serve immediately.

Nutritional value: (per serving)
- Calories: 350
- Fat: 10g
- Protein: 15g
- Carbohydrates: 50g
- Fiber: 5g
- Sugar: 15g
- Cooking time: 5 minutes

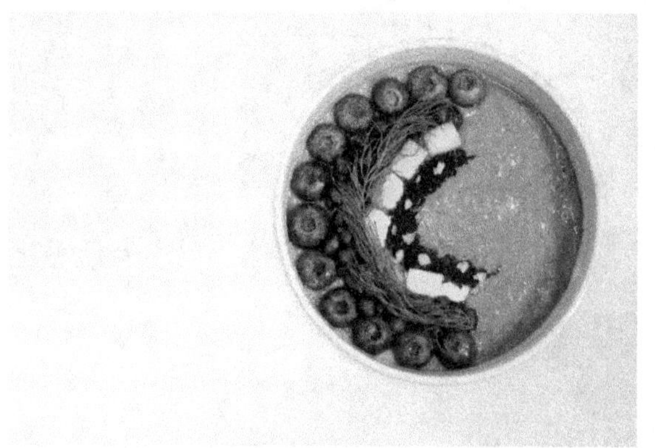

<u>**Berry and Kale Smoothie Bowl**</u>

Ingredients:
- One cup frozen berries
- Half cup kale, chopped
- One cup milk or yogurt
- One banana, sliced

- One tablespoon chia seeds (optional)

Preparation:
- Combine all of the ingredients in a blender and blend until smooth.
- Pour the smoothie into a bowl and top with additional berries, granola, and chia seeds (if desired).
- Serve immediately.

Nutritional value: (per serving)
- Calories: 300
- Fat: 5g
- Protein: 10g
- Carbohydrates: 50g
- Fiber: 10g
- Sugar: 15g

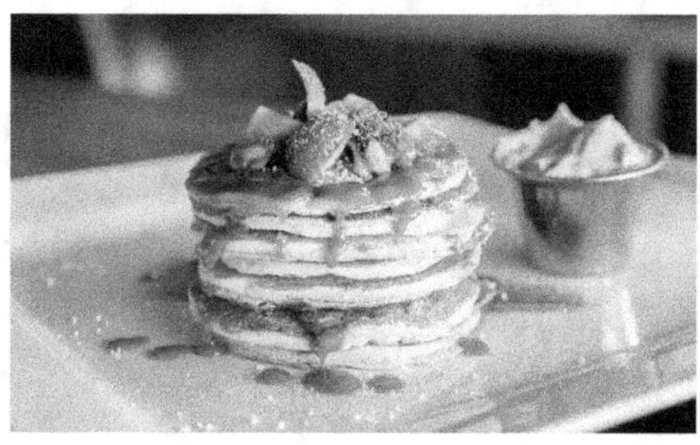

Whole-Grain Pancakes with Fruit

Ingredients:

- One cup whole-wheat flour
- One tablespoon sugar1 teaspoon baking powder
- Half teaspoon baking soda
- One quarter teaspoon salt
- One cup milk
- One egg
- One tablespoon vegetable oil
- One quarter teaspoon vanilla extract
- Half cup fruit, chopped (such as blueberries, strawberries, or bananas)

Preparation:

- In a large bowl, whisk together the flour, sugar, baking powder, baking soda, and salt.
- In a separate bowl, whisk together the milk, egg, oil, and vanilla extract.
- Add the wet ingredients to the dry ingredients and whisk until just combined. Do not overmix.

- Heat a griddle or large skillet over medium heat. Grease the griddle with butter or cooking spray.
- Pour 1/4 cup of batter onto the hot griddle for each pancake.
- Cook for 2-3 minutes per side, or until golden brown and cooked through.
- Serve immediately with your favourite fresh fruit.

Nutritional value: (per serving)
- Calories: 250
- Fat: 5g
- Protein: 10g
- Carbohydrates: 40g
- Fiber: 5g
- Sugar: 10g
- Cooking time: 10-12 minutes

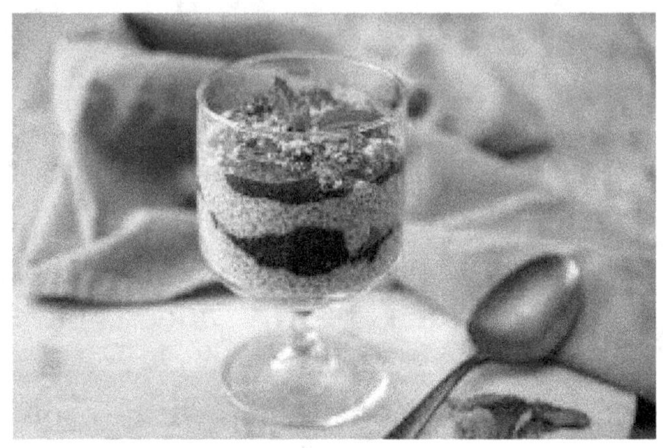

Chia Seed Pudding

Ingredients:

- Two tablespoons chia seeds
- One cup almond milk (unsweetened)
- Half teaspoon vanilla extract
- Half cup fresh mixed berries

Preparation:

- In a jar or bowl, mix chia seeds, almond milk, and vanilla extract.
- Stir well and refrigerate for a few hours or overnight until it thickens.
- Serve with fresh mixed berries.

Nutritional Value:

- Calories: 220
- Protein: 6g
- Fiber: 10g
- Healthy Fats: 7g
- Cooking Time: 5 minutes (plus chilling time)

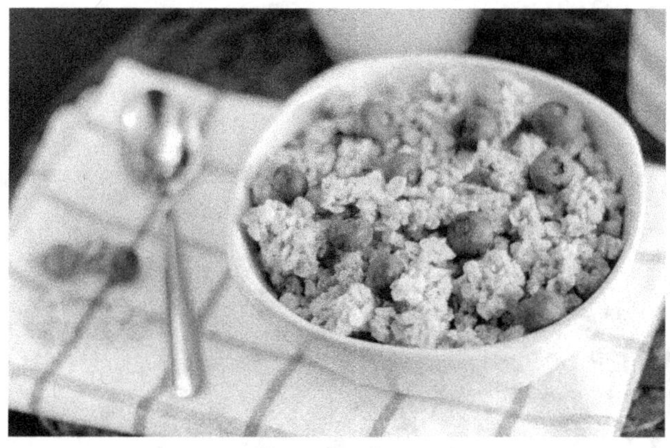

Quinoa Breakfast Bowl

Ingredients:

- Half cup cooked quinoa
- One quarter cup almond milk (unsweetened)
- One quarter teaspoon cinnamon
- Half medium apple, chopped
- One tablespoon chopped nuts (e.g., walnuts or almonds)

Preparation:
- Combine cooked quinoa, almond milk, and cinnamon in a saucepan. Heat over low heat until warmed.
- Top with chopped apple and nuts.

Nutritional Value:
- Calories: 280
- Protein: 6g
- Fiber: 5g
- Healthy Fats: 7g
- Cooking Time: 10 minutes

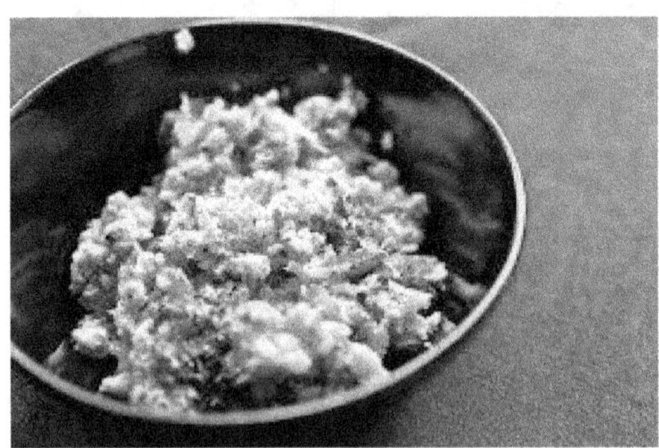

Veggie Scramble

Ingredients:
- Two large eggs

- One quarter cup diced bell peppers (various colors)
- One quarter cup diced tomatoes
- Half tablespoons diced onions
- Salt and pepper to taste
- Cooking spray

Preparation:
- Heat a non-stick skillet over medium heat and coat with cooking spray.
- Add diced onions and bell peppers and cook until slightly softened.
- Whisk the eggs with salt and pepper and pour them into the skillet.
- Stir until the eggs are scrambled and cooked to your preference. Add diced tomatoes.

Nutritional Value:
- Calories: 190
- Protein: 12g
- Fibre: 2g
- Healthy Fats: 10g
- Cooking Time: 10 minutes

These heart-healthy breakfast recipes are not only delicious but also nutritious, providing a well-rounded start to your day while supporting your cardiovascular health. Adjust portion sizes and ingredients to meet your specific dietary needs and preferences. Enjoy a heart-healthy breakfast for a nourishing start to your day!

CHAPTER 5

Delicious Lunch Recipes

This cookbook offers a delectable array of lunch options that not only tickle your taste buds but also prioritise the well-being of your heart.

With an emphasis on heart-healthy ingredients, these dishes are designed to reduce your risk of heart disease while delighting your palate. Make your lunchtime a celebration of good health and savour the path to a stronger, happier heart with our delicious lunch recipes.

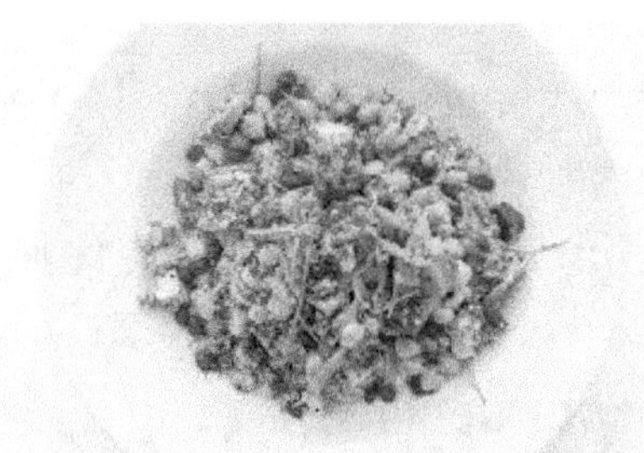

Lentil Salad with Avocado and Lemon Vinaigrette

Ingredients:
- 1 cup cooked lentils
- 1/2 avocado, diced
- 1/4 cup chopped cucumber
- 1/4 cup chopped red onion
- 1/4 cup chopped fresh herbs (such as parsley, cilantro, or basil)
- 2 tablespoons lemon juice
- 1 tablespoon olive oil
- Salt and pepper to taste

Preparation:
- Combine the lentils, avocado, cucumber, red onion, and herbs in a bowl.
- In a separate bowl, whisk together the lemon juice, olive oil, salt, and pepper.
- Pour the vinaigrette over the lentil salad and toss to coat.
- Serve immediately or chill for later.

Nutritional value: (per serving)
- Calories: 300
- Fat: 10g
- Protein: 15g

- Carbohydrates: 30g
- Fiber: 10g
- Sugar: 5g
- Cooking time: 10 minutes

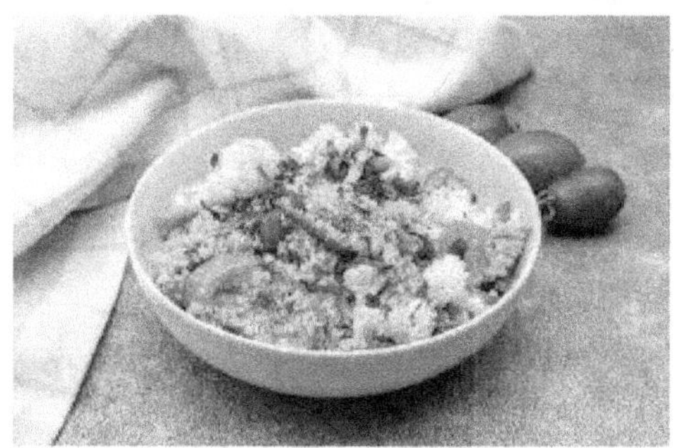

Quinoa Salad with Chickpeas and Roasted Vegetables

Ingredients:
- 1 cup cooked quinoa
- 1/2 cup cooked chickpeas
- 1/2 cup roasted vegetables (such as broccoli, carrots, and zucchini)
- 1/4 cup chopped red onion
- 1/4 cup chopped fresh herbs (such as parsley, cilantro, or basil)
- 2 tablespoons olive oil
- 1 tablespoon lemon juice
- Salt and pepper to taste

Preparation:

- Combine the quinoa, chickpeas, roasted vegetables, red onion, and herbs in a bowl.
- In a separate bowl, whisk together the olive oil, lemon juice, salt, and pepper.
- Pour the vinaigrette over the quinoa salad and toss to coat.
- Serve immediately or chill for later.

Nutritional value: (per serving)

- Calories: 350
- Fat: 10g
- Protein: 15g
- Carbohydrates: 45g
- Fiber: 10gSugar: 5g
- Cooking time: 15 minutes

Salmon Salad Sandwich on Whole-Wheat Bread

Ingredients:

- 2 slices whole-wheat bread
- 1/4 cup canned salmon, drained

- 1 tablespoon mayonnaise
- 1/4 cup chopped celery
- 1 tablespoon chopped red onion
- 1/4 teaspoon lemon juice
- Salt and pepper to taste

Preparation:
- Combine the salmon, mayonnaise, celery, red onion, lemon juice, salt, and pepper in a bowl.
- Spread the salmon salad on the bread slices.
- Sandwich the bread slices together and cut in half.
- Serve immediately.

Nutritional value: (per serving)
- Calories: 250
- Fat: 10g
- Protein: 15g
- Carbohydrates: 30g
- Fiber: 5g
- Sugar: 2g
- Cooking time: 10 minutes

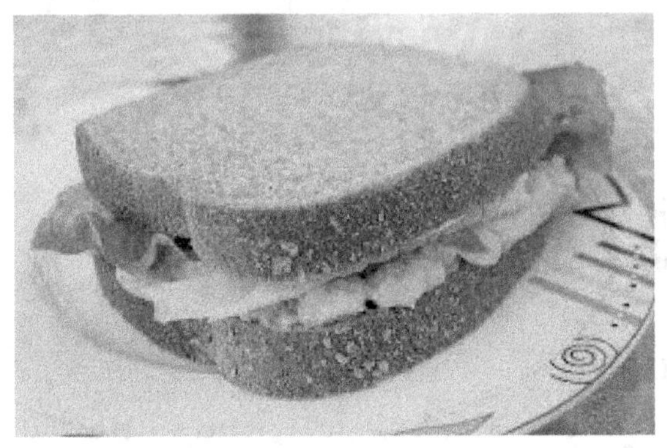

Tuna Salad Sandwich on Whole-Wheat Bread

Ingredients:

- 2 slices whole-wheat bread
- 1/4 cup canned tuna, drained
- 1 tablespoon mayonnaise
- 1/4 cup chopped celery
- 1 tablespoon chopped red onion
- 1/4 teaspoon lemon juice
- Salt and pepper to taste

Preparation:

- Combine the tuna, mayonnaise, celery, red onion, lemon juice, salt, and pepper in a bowl.
- Spread the tuna salad on the bread slices.

- Sandwich the bread slices together and cut in half.
- Serve immediately.

Nutritional value: (per serving)
- Calories: 250
- Fat: 10g
- Protein: 15g
- Carbohydrates: 30g
- Fiber: 5g
- Sugar: 2g
- Cooking time: 10 minutes

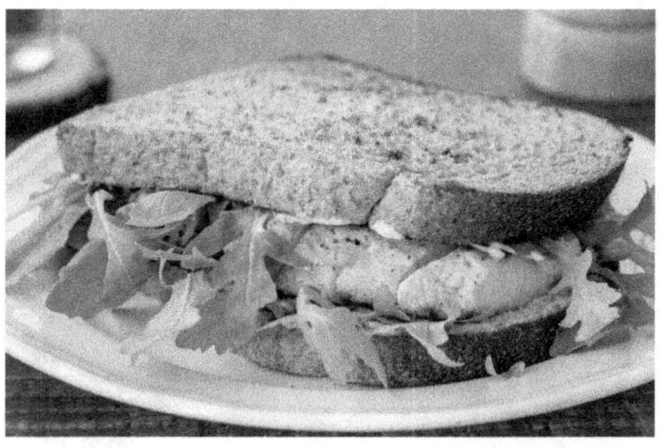

Chicken Salad Sandwich on Whole-Wheat Bread

Ingredients:
- 2 slices whole-wheat bread

- 1/4 cup cooked chicken, chopped
- 1 tablespoon mayonnaise
- 1/4 cup chopped celery
- 1 tablespoon chopped red onion
- 1/4 teaspoon lemon juice
- Salt and pepper to taste

Preparation:

- Combine the chicken, mayonnaise, celery, red onion, lemon juice, salt, and pepper in a bowl.
- Spread the chicken salad on the bread slices.
- Sandwich the bread slices together and cut in half.
- Serve immediately.

Nutritional value: (per serving)

- Calories: 250
- Fat: 10g
- Protein: 15g
- Carbohydrates: 30g
- Fiber: 5g
- Sugar: 2g
- Cooking time: 10 minutes

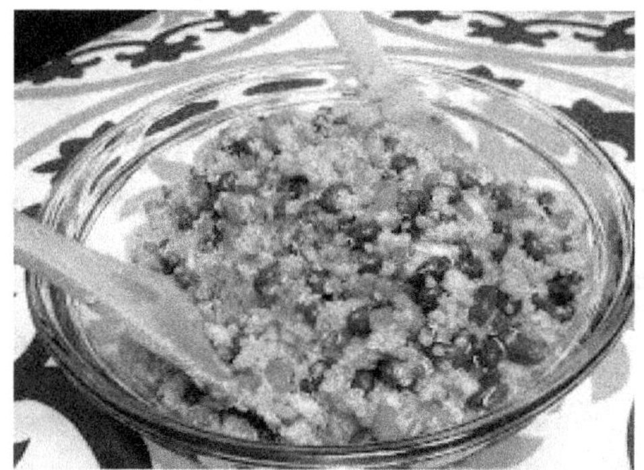

Quinoa and Black Bean Salad

Ingredients:
- 1 cup cooked quinoa
- 1/2 cup black beans, rinsed and drained
- 1/4 cup chopped red onion
- 1/4 cup chopped cilantro
- 2 tablespoons olive oil
- 1 tablespoon lemon juice
- 1/2 teaspoon salt
- 1/4 teaspoon black pepper

Preparation:
- In a large bowl, combine the quinoa, black beans, red onion, and cilantro.
- In a small bowl, whisk together the olive oil, lemon juice, salt, and pepper.

- Pour the vinaigrette over the quinoa salad and toss to coat.
- Serve immediately or chill for later.

Nutritional value: (per serving)
- Calories: 250
- Fat: 10g
- Protein: 10g
- Carbohydrates: 35g
- Fiber: 5g
- Sugar: 5g
- Cooking time: 15 minutes

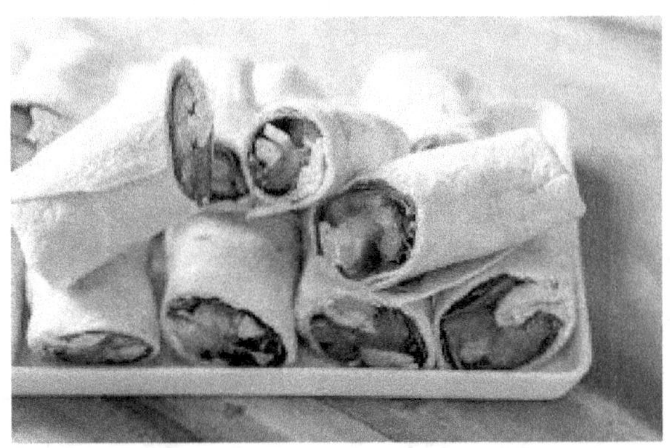

Grilled Chicken and Vegetable Wrap

Ingredients:
- 1 whole-wheat tortilla
- 1/4 cup cooked chicken, shredded

- 1/4 cup grilled vegetables (such as zucchini, carrots, and bell peppers)
- 1 tablespoon hummus
- 1/4 teaspoon salt
- 1/4 teaspoon black pepper

Preparation:
- Spread the hummus on the tortilla.
- Top with the chicken, grilled vegetables, salt, and pepper.
- Roll up the tortilla tightly and cut in half.
- Serve immediately.

Nutritional value: (per serving)
- Calories: 250
- Fat: 5g
- Protein: 20g
- Carbohydrates: 30g
- Fiber: 5g
- Sugar: 5g
- Cooking time: 10 minutes

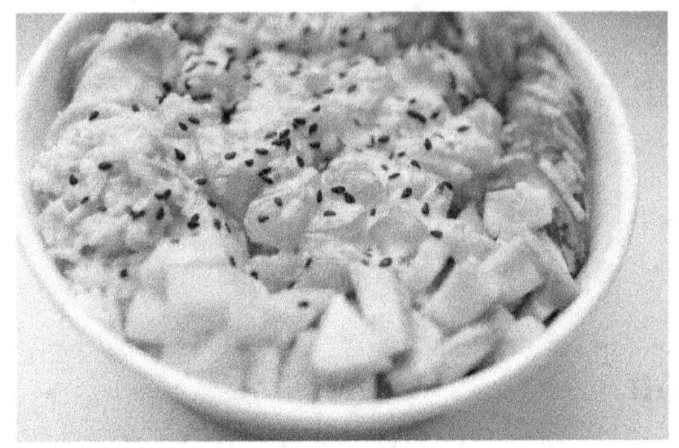

Salmon and Quinoa Bowl

Ingredients:

- 1 cup cooked quinoa
- 1/4 pound salmon fillet, grilled or baked
- 1/2 cup roasted vegetables (such as broccoli, carrots, and zucchini)
- 1/4 cup chopped red onion
- 2 tablespoons avocado oil
- 1 tablespoon lemon juice
- 1/4 teaspoon salt
- 1/4 teaspoon black pepper

Preparation:

- In a bowl, combine the quinoa, salmon, roasted vegetables, red onion, avocado oil, lemon juice, salt, and pepper.

- Toss to coat.Serve immediately.

Nutritional value: (per serving)
- Calories: 400
- Fat: 15g
- Protein: 30g
- Carbohydrates: 40g
- Fiber: 5g
- Sugar: 5g
- Cooking time: 20 minutes

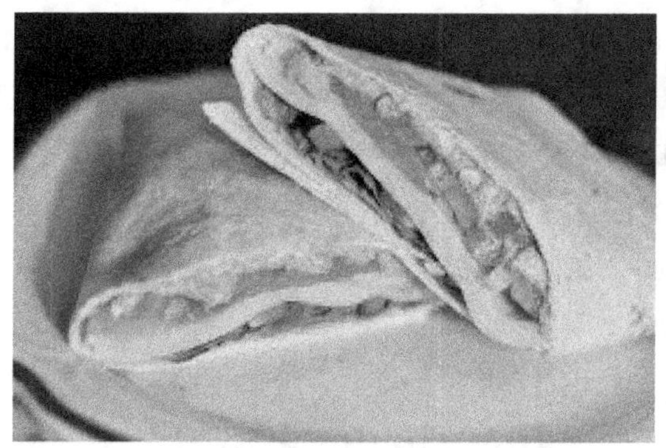

Turkey and Avocado Wrap

Ingredients:
- 1 whole-wheat tortilla
- 1/4 cup cooked turkey, sliced
- 1/4 avocado, mashed
- 1 tablespoon Dijon mustard

- 1/4 teaspoon salt
- 1/4 teaspoon black pepper

Preparation:
- Spread the Dijon mustard on the tortilla.
- Top with the turkey, avocado, salt, and pepper.
- Roll up the tortilla tightly and cut in half.Serve immediately.

Nutritional value: (per serving)
- Calories: 250
- Fat: 10g
- Protein: 20g
- Carbohydrates: 30g
- Fiber: 5g
- Sugar: 5g
- Cooking time: 10 minutes

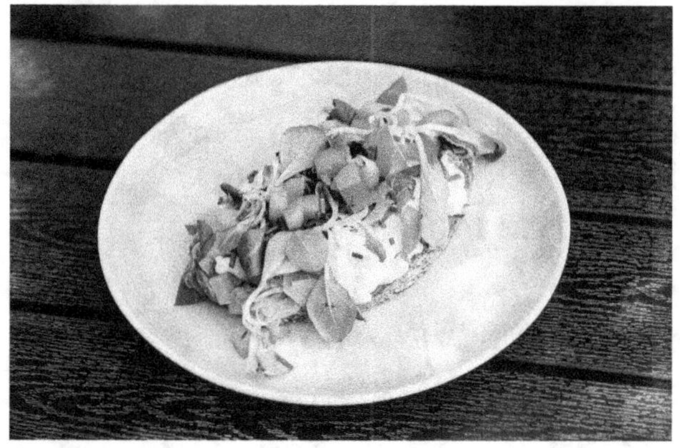

<u>**Spinach and Strawberry Salad**</u>

Ingredients:
- 4 cups baby spinach
- 1 cup strawberries, sliced
- 1/4 cup crumbled feta cheese
- 2 tablespoons olive oil
- 1 tablespoon balsamic vinegar
- 1/4 teaspoon salt
- 1/4 teaspoon black pepper

Preparation:
- In a large bowl, combine the spinach, strawberries, and feta cheese.
- In a small bowl, whisk together the olive oil, balsamic vinegar, salt, and pepper.

- Pour the dressing over the salad and toss to coat.Serve immediately.

Nutritional value: (per serving)
- Calories: 150
- Fat: 10g
- Protein: 5g
- Carbohydrates: 15g
- Fiber: 5g
- Sugar: 10g
- Cooking time: 5 minutes

These heart-healthy lunch recipes are packed with nutrients and flavor, making them a delicious and nutritious choice for supporting your cardiovascular health. Adjust portion sizes and ingredients to meet your specific dietary needs and preferences. Enjoy a nourishing and satisfying lunch!

CHAPTER 6

Flavourful Dinner Recipes

This cookbook offers an enticing array of dinner options that not only tantalise your taste buds but also prioritise your heart's well-being. Our recipes are thoughtfully crafted to be both delicious and nutritious, with a focus on heart-healthy ingredients.

By choosing these dishes, you're taking a step towards reducing the risk of heart disease while relishing every bite. Begin your journey to a healthier heart with our flavour-packed dinner recipes.

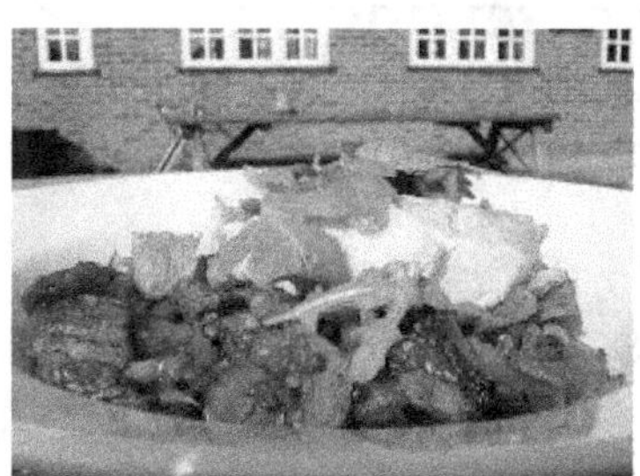

Grilled Salmon with Roasted Vegetables

Ingredients:
- 1 pound salmon fillet
- 1 tablespoon olive oil
- 1/2 teaspoon salt
- 1/4 teaspoon black pepper
- 2 cups roasted vegetables (such as broccoli, carrots, and zucchini)

Preparation:
- Preheat grill to medium heat.Brush the salmon fillet with olive oil and season with salt and pepper.
- Grill the salmon for 6-8 minutes per side, or until cooked through.
- Serve the salmon with the roasted vegetables.

Nutritional value: (per serving)
- Calories: 400
- Fat: 15g
- Protein: 30g
- Carbohydrates: 40g
- Fiber: 5g
- Sugar: 5g
- Cooking time: 20 minutes

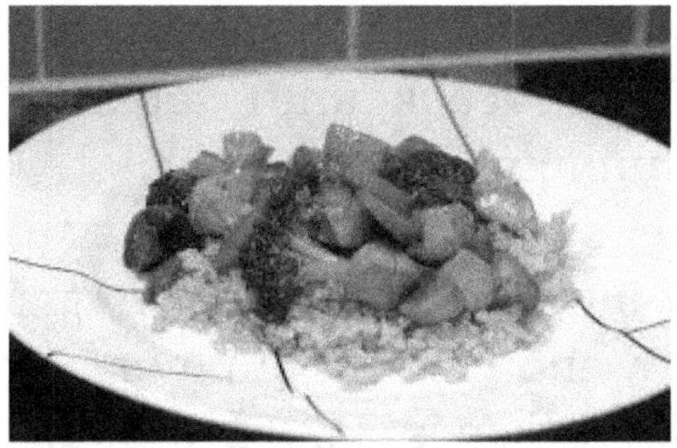

Chicken Stir-Fry with Brown Rice

Ingredients:
- 1 tablespoon olive oil
- 1 pound chicken breast, cut into bite-sized pieces
- 1 onion, chopped
- 2 bell peppers, chopped
- 1 cup broccoli, chopped
- 1/2 cup soy sauce
- 1/4 cup rice vinegar
- 1 tablespoon sesame oil
- 1/4 teaspoon black pepper
- 2 cups cooked brown rice

Preparation:
- Heat the olive oil in a large skillet or wok over medium-high heat.
- Add the chicken and cook until browned, about 5 minutes.

- Add the onion, bell peppers, and broccoli and cook until softened, about 5 minutes.
- Add the soy sauce, rice vinegar, sesame oil, and black pepper and cook for another 1-2 minutes, or until the chicken is cooked through.
- Serve over brown rice.

Nutritional value: (per serving)
- Calories: 450
- Fat: 10g
- Protein: 40g
- Carbohydrates: 60g
- Fiber: 10g
- Sugar: 10g
- Cooking time: 20 minutes

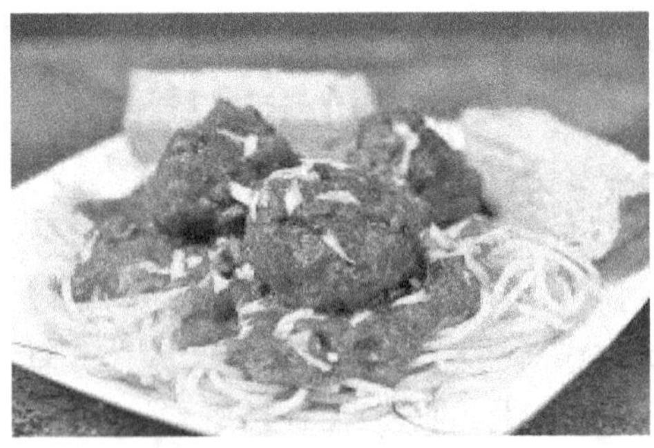

Spaghetti with Meatballs

Ingredients:

- 1 pound ground beef
- 1/2 cup bread crumbs
- 1/4 cup grated Parmesan cheese
- 1 egg
- 1/4 cup chopped onion
- 1/4 cup chopped parsley
- 1 teaspoon garlic powder
- 1/2 teaspoon salt
- 1/4 teaspoon black pepper
- 1 (28 ounce) can crushed tomatoes
- 1 pound spaghetti

Preparation:

- Preheat oven to 350 degrees F (175 degrees C).
- In a large bowl, combine the ground beef, bread crumbs, Parmesan cheese, egg, onion, parsley, garlic powder, salt, and pepper. Mix well.
- Form the meat mixture into small meatballs.
- Place the meatballs on a baking sheet and bake for 20-25 minutes, or until cooked through.

- Meanwhile, cook the spaghetti according to package directions.
- Drain the spaghetti and return it to the pot.
- Add the meatballs and crushed tomatoes to the spaghetti and stir to combine.Serve immediately.

Nutritional value: (per serving)
- Calories: 550
- Fat: 20g
- Protein: 35g
- Carbohydrates: 70g
- Fiber: 5g
- Sugar: 10g
- Cooking time: 45 minutes

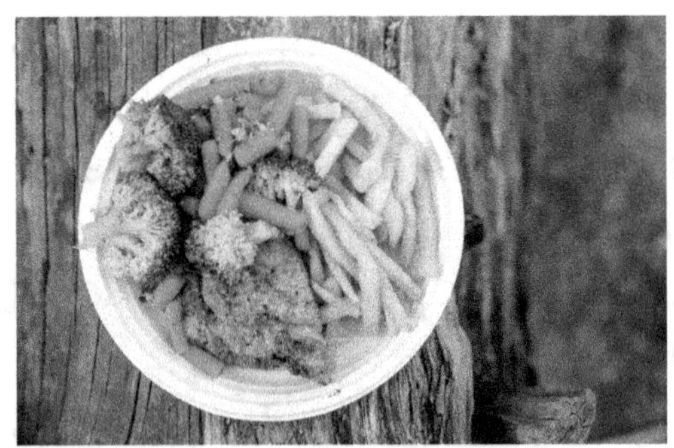

Grilled Chicken Breast with Roasted Potatoes and Broccoli

Ingredients:

- 2 boneless, skinless chicken breasts
- 1 tablespoon olive oil
- 1/2 teaspoon salt
- 1/4 teaspoon black pepper
- 1 pound potatoes, peeled and cut into bite-sized pieces
- 1 head of broccoli, cut into florets
- 2 tablespoons olive oil
- 1/2 teaspoon salt
- 1/4 teaspoon black pepper

Preparation:

- Preheat grill to medium heat.
- Brush the chicken breasts with olive oil and season with salt and pepper.
- Grill the chicken breasts for 6-8 minutes per side, or until cooked through.
- Meanwhile, preheat oven to 400 degrees F (200 degrees C).
- Toss the potatoes and broccoli with olive oil, salt, and pepper.
- Spread the potatoes and broccoli on a baking sheet and roast for 20-25 minutes, or until tender.

- Serve the grilled chicken breasts with the roasted potatoes and broccoli.

Nutritional value: (per serving)
- Calories: 400
- Fat: 10g
- Protein: 40g
- Carbohydrates: 40g
- Fiber: 5g
- Sugar: 5g
- Cooking time: 45 minutes

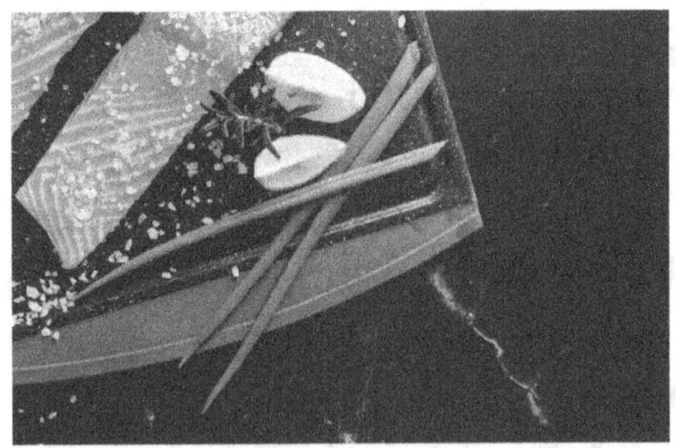

Baked Salmon with Asparagus

Ingredients:
- 1 salmon fillet (about 6 ounces)
- 1 tablespoon olive oil
- 1/4 teaspoon salt

- 1/4 teaspoon black pepper
- 1/2 cup asparagus florets

Preparation:
- Preheat oven to 400 degrees F (200 degrees C).
- Place the salmon fillet on a baking sheet.
- Drizzle with olive oil and season with salt and pepper.
- Surround the salmon with the asparagus florets.
- Bake for 12-15 minutes, or until the salmon is cooked through and the asparagus is tender.

Nutritional value: (per serving)
- Calories: 300
- Fat: 15g
- Protein: 30g
- Carbohydrates: 10g
- Fiber: 5g
- Sugar: 5g
- Cooking time: 20 minutes

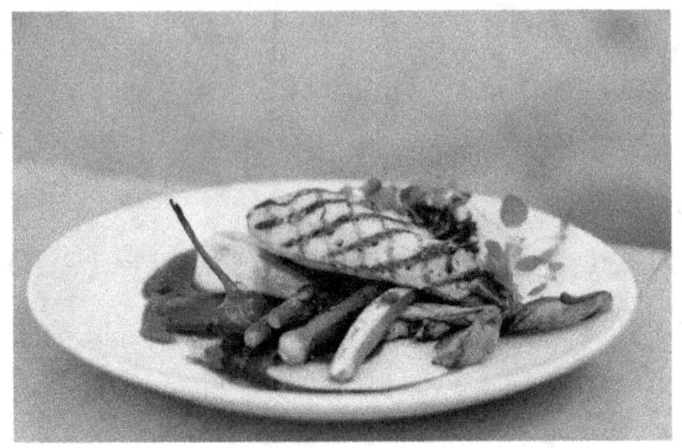

Lemon Herb Grilled Chicken

Ingredients:

- 4 boneless, skinless chicken breasts
- 1/4 cup olive oil
- 1/4 cup lemon juice1 teaspoon garlic powder
- 1/2 teaspoon dried oregano
- 1/4 teaspoon salt
- 1/4 teaspoon black pepper

Preparation:

- In a large bowl, combine the chicken breasts, olive oil, lemon juice, garlic powder, oregano, salt, and pepper.
- Toss to coat.
- Cover the bowl and refrigerate for at least 30 minutes, or up to overnight.
- Preheat grill to medium heat.

- Grill the chicken breasts for 6-8 minutes per side, or until cooked through.Serve immediately.

Nutritional value: (per serving)
- Calories: 250
- Fat: 5g
- Protein: 40g
- Carbohydrates: 5g
- Fiber: 1g
- Sugar: 1g
- Cooking time: 15 minutes

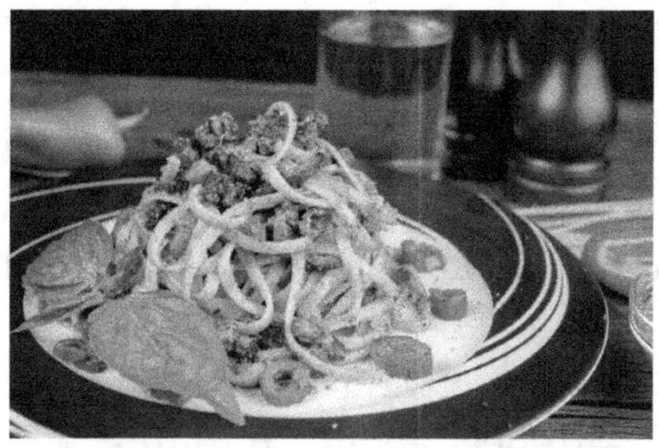

Spaghetti Squash with Tomato and Basil

Ingredients:
- 1 spaghetti squash

- 1 tablespoon olive oil
- 1/2 onion, chopped
- 2 cloves garlic, minced
- 1 (14.5 ounce) can diced tomatoes, undrained
- 1/4 cup chopped fresh basil
- 1/4 teaspoon salt
- 1/4 teaspoon black pepper

Preparation:
- Preheat oven to 400 degrees F (200 degrees C).
- Cut the spaghetti squash in half lengthwise and remove the seeds.
- Place the spaghetti squash halves on a baking sheet and bake for 45 minutes, or until tender.
- Meanwhile, heat the olive oil in a large saucepan over medium heat.
- Add the onion and garlic and cook until softened, about 5 minutes.
- Add the diced tomatoes, basil, salt, and pepper and cook for an additional 10 minutes, or until the sauce has thickened.

- Once the spaghetti squash is tender, use a fork to scrape the flesh into strands.
- Top the spaghetti squash with the tomato sauce and serve immediately.

Nutritional value: (per serving)
- Calories: 200
- Fat: 5g
- Protein: 10g
- Carbohydrates: 35g
- Fiber: 10g
- Sugar: 10g
- Cooking time: 55 minutes

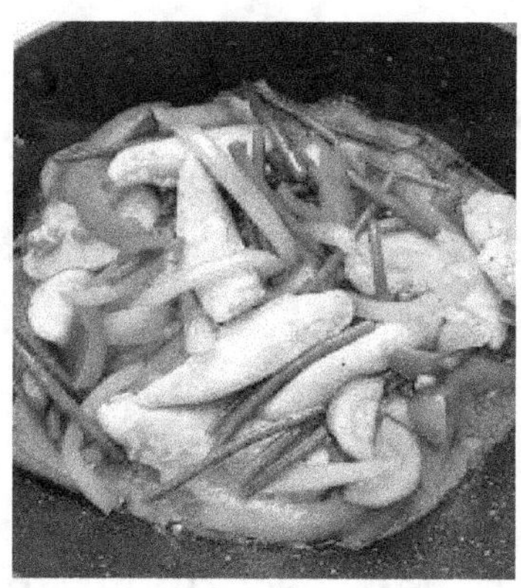

Portobello Mushroom Fajitas

Ingredients:

- 2 portobello mushrooms, stemmed and sliced
- 1 tablespoon olive oil
- 1/2 onion, chopped
- 1 bell pepper, chopped
- 1 teaspoon chili powder
- 1/2 teaspoon cumin
- 1/4 teaspoon salt
- 1/4 teaspoon black pepper6 (8-inch) tortillas
- Your favorite fajita toppings (such as guacamole, sour cream, salsa, and cheese)

Preparation:

- Heat the olive oil in a large skillet over medium heat.
- Add the mushrooms, onion, and bell pepper and cook until softened, about 10 minutes.
- Sprinkle with the chili powder, cumin, salt, and pepper and cook for an additional 1 minute.
- Warm the tortillas according to package directions.

- Divide the mushroom fajita mixture evenly among the tortillas and top with your favourite fajita toppings.Serve immediately.

Nutritional value: (per serving)
- Calories: 250
- Fat: 10g
- Protein: 15g
- Carbohydrates: 35g
- Fiber: 10g
- Sugar: 5kg

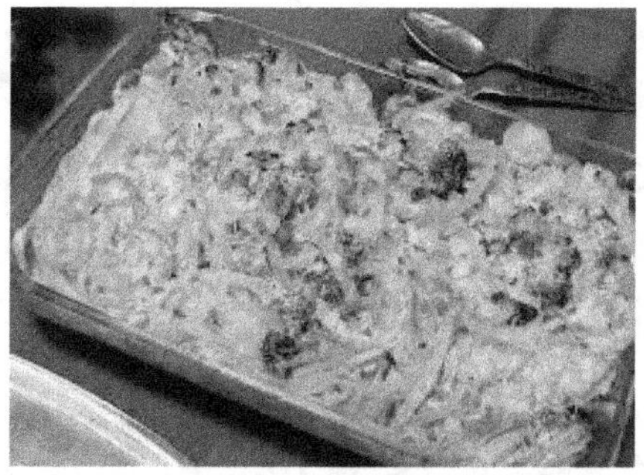

Lemon Garlic Shrimp and Broccoli

Ingredients:
- 1 pound shrimp, peeled and deveined
- 1 tablespoon olive oil

- 1/4 cup lemon juice
- 2 cloves garlic, minced
- 1/4 teaspoon salt
- 1/4 teaspoon black pepper
- 1 head of broccoli, cut into florets

Preparation:
- Heat the olive oil in a large skillet over medium heat.
- Add the shrimp and cook until pink and cooked through, about 3 minutes per side.
- Add the lemon juice, garlic, salt, and pepper to the skillet and stir to combine.
- Add the broccoli to the skillet and cook until tender, about 5 minutes.Serve immediately.

Nutritional value: (per serving)
- Calories: 200
- Fat: 5g
- Protein: 30g
- Carbohydrates: 10g
- Fiber: 5gSugar: 5g
- Cooking time: 15 minutes

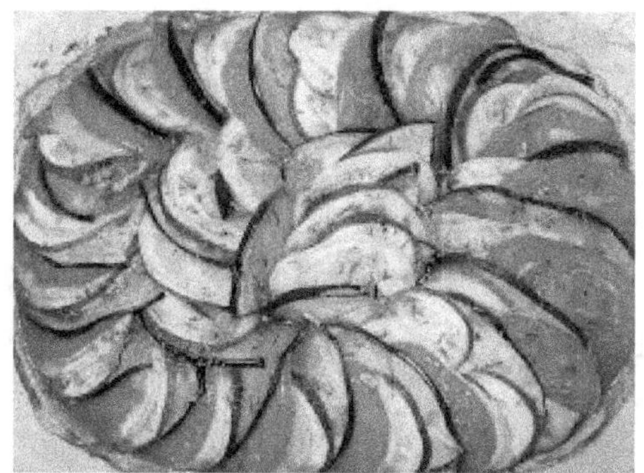

Eggplant and Zucchini Ratatouille

Ingredients:

- 1 tablespoon olive oil
- 1 onion, chopped
- 2 cloves garlic, minced
- 1 eggplant, diced
- 2 zucchini, diced
- 1 (14.5 ounce) can diced tomatoes, undrained
- 1/2 cup chopped fresh basil
- 1/4 teaspoon salt
- 1/4 teaspoon black pepper

Preparation:

- Heat the olive oil in a large pot over medium heat.
- Add the onion and garlic and cook until softened, about 5 minutes.

- Add the eggplant, zucchini, diced tomatoes, basil, salt, and pepper to the pot and stir to combine.
- Bring to a boil, then reduce heat to low and simmer for 20-25 minutes, or until the vegetables are tender.

Nutritional value: (per serving)
- Calories: 150
- Fat: 5g
- Protein: 5g
- Carbohydrates: 25g
- Fiber: 10g
- Sugar: 5g
- Cooking time: 30 minutes

These heart-healthy dinner recipes are not only delicious but also packed with nutrients, making them a fantastic choice for supporting your cardiovascular health. Adjust portion sizes and ingredients to meet your specific dietary needs and preferences. Enjoy a nourishing and satisfying dinner!

CHAPTER 7

Nourishing Smoothie Recipes

Introducing "Smoothie Recipes for Heart Disease" – a refreshing approach to supporting your cardiovascular health. Each smoothie combines heart-healthy ingredients in a delightful blend that makes it easy to prioritise your cardiovascular well-being. Our smoothies are a perfect combination of health and taste, making it simpler than ever to embark on a heart-healthy journey.

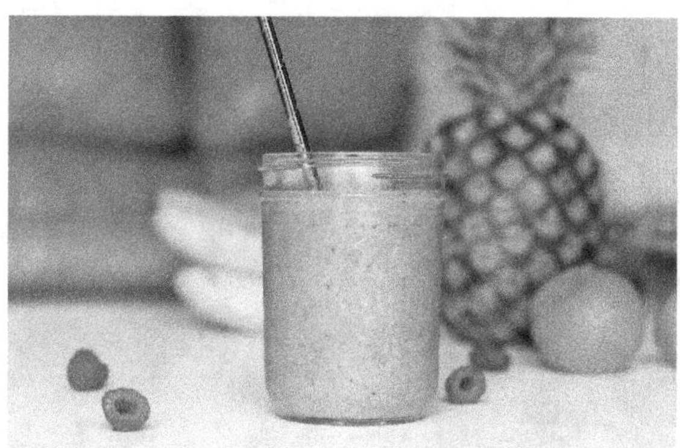

Berry Blast Smoothie

Ingredients:

- 1 cup mixed berries (e.g., strawberries, blueberries, raspberries)
- 1/2 banana
- 1/2 cup Greek yogurt (low-fat)
- 1/2 cup spinach leaves
- 1/2 cup almond milk (unsweetened)
- 1 tablespoon chia seeds

Preparation:

- Blend mixed berries, banana, Greek yoghurt, spinach, and almond milk until smooth.
- Add chia seeds and blend for a few more seconds.

Nutritional Value:

- Calories: 250
- Protein: 10g
- Fibre: 8g
- Healthy Fats: 5g
- Preparation Time: 5 minutes

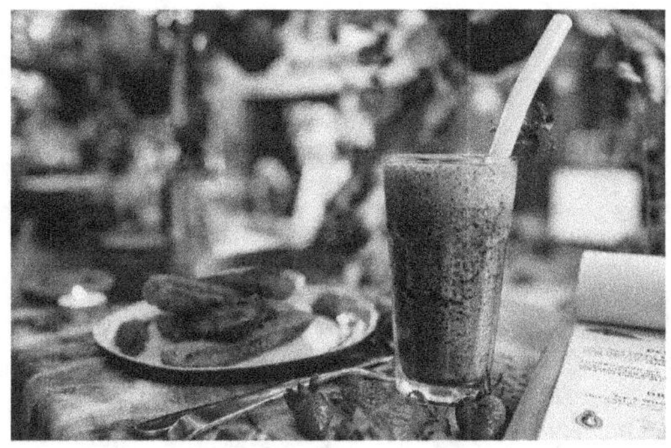

Pomegranate Blueberry Bliss

Ingredients:
- 1/2 cup pomegranate seeds
- 1/2 cup blueberries
- 1/2 cup Greek yoghurt (low-fat)
- 1/2 cup almond milk (unsweetened)
- 1 tablespoon hemp seeds

Preparation:
- Blend pomegranate seeds, blueberries, Greek yoghurt, and almond milk until smooth.
- Add hemp seeds and blend for a few more seconds.

Nutritional Value:
- Calories: 250
- Protein: 9g

- Fibre: 6g
- Healthy Fats: 5g
- Preparation Time: 5 minutes

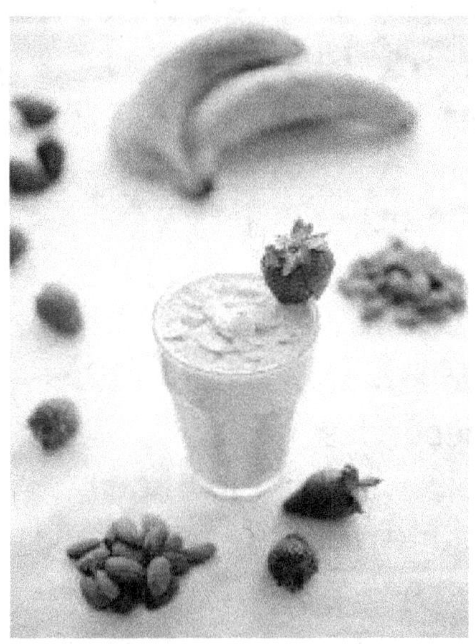

<u>Banana Almond Smoothie</u>

Ingredients:
- 1 banana
- 1/4 cup almond butter
- 1/2 cup almond milk (unsweetened)
- 1/2 cup Greek yoghurt (low-fat)
- 1/2 teaspoon cinnamon
- 1/2 teaspoon vanilla extract

Preparation:

- Blend banana, almond butter, almond milk, Greek yoghurt, cinnamon, and vanilla extract until smooth.

Nutritional Value:

- Calories: 340
- Protein: 10g
- Fiber: 6g
- Healthy Fats: 20g
- Preparation Time: 5 minutes

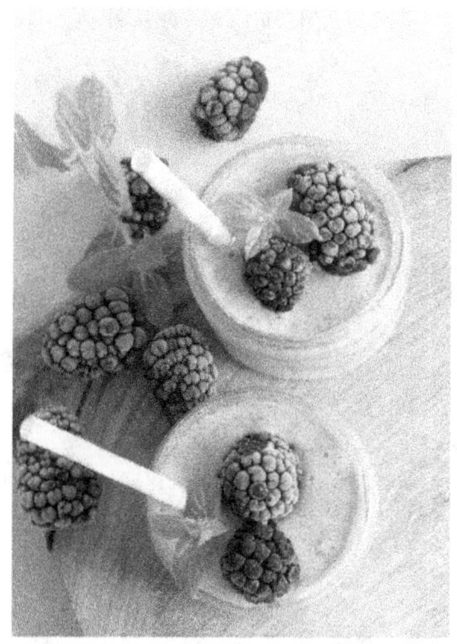

Beet and Berry Smoothie

Ingredients:

- 1 small cooked beet (peeled and diced)
- 1/2 cup mixed berries (e.g., raspberries, blackberries)
- 1/2 cup Greek yoghurt (low-fat)
- 1/2 cup water
- 1 tablespoon honey (optional)

Preparation:

- Blend cooked beet, mixed berries, Greek yoghurt, and water until smooth.
- Add honey for added sweetness if desired.

Nutritional Value:

- Calories: 200
- Protein: 8g
- Fiber: 6g
- Healthy Fats: 2g
- Preparation Time: 5 minutes

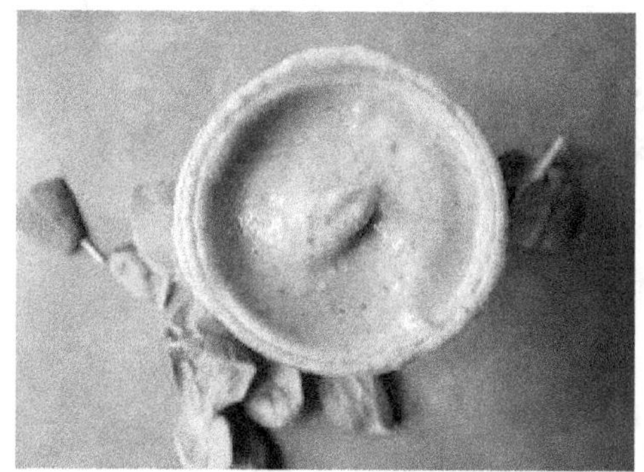

Avocado Spinach Smoothie

Ingredients:
- 1/2 avocado
- 1 cup spinach leaves
- 1/2 cup banana
- 1/2 cup almond milk (unsweetened)
- 1/2 cup Greek yoghurt (low-fat)
- 1 tablespoon flax seeds

Preparation:
- Blend avocado, spinach, banana, almond milk, and Greek yoghurt until smooth.
- Add flaxseeds and blend for a few more seconds.

Nutritional Value:
- Calories: 280

- Protein: 9g
- Fibre: 8g
- Healthy Fats: 12g
- Preparation Time: 5 minutes

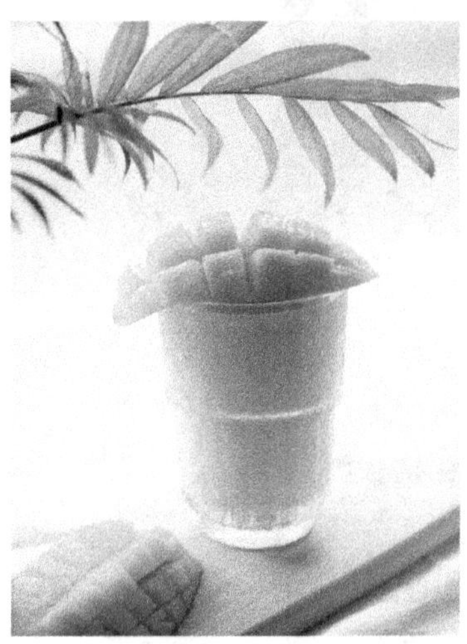

Pineapple Mango Protein Smoothie

Ingredients:
- 1/2 cup pineapple chunks
- 1/2 cup mango chunks
- 1 cup almond milk (unsweetened)
- 1 scoop vanilla protein powder
- 1 tablespoon chia seeds

Preparation:
- Blend pineapple, mango, almond milk, vanilla protein powder, and chia seeds until smooth.

Nutritional Value:
- Calories: 280
- Protein: 15g
- Fiber: 7g
- Healthy Fats: 7g
- Preparation Time: 5 minutes

These heart-healthy smoothie recipes are not only delicious but also packed with nutrients, making them a great choice for supporting your cardiovascular health. Adjust portion sizes and ingredients to meet your specific dietary needs and preferences. Enjoy a refreshing and nutritious smoothie!

CHAPTER 8

Mindful Snacks Recipes

Snack Recipes for Heart Disease" offers a delightful selection of heart-healthy snacks that prove you don't have to compromise on taste to support your cardiovascular well-being. With these easy-to-prepare recipes, you can curb your cravings while reducing your risk of heart disease. Enjoy every bite with the confidence that you're making a positive difference in your life and well-being.

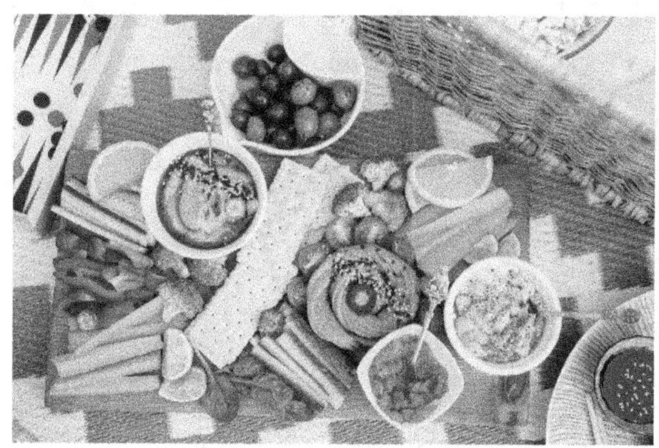

Hummus and Veggie Platter

Ingredients:

- 1/2 cup hummus
- Baby carrots
- Cucumber slices
- Cherry tomatoes

Preparation:

- Arrange baby carrots, cucumber slices, and cherry tomatoes on a platter.
- Serve with a side of hummus for dipping.

Nutritional Value:

- Calories: 150
- Protein: 4g
- Fiber: 5g
- Healthy Fats: 7g
- Preparation Time: 5 minutes

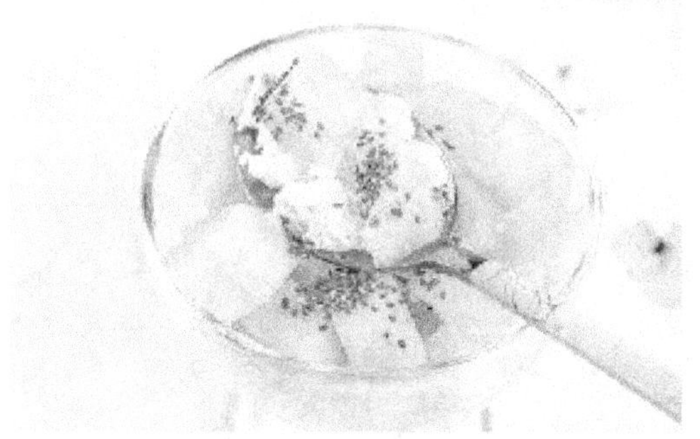

Cottage Cheese and Pineapple

Ingredients:
- 1/2 cup low-fat cottage cheese
- 1/2 cup fresh pineapple chunks

Preparation:
- Top low-fat cottage cheese with fresh pineapple chunks.

Nutritional Value:
- Calories: 180
- Protein: 14g
- Fiber: 2g
- Healthy Fats: 1g
- Preparation Time: 2 minutes

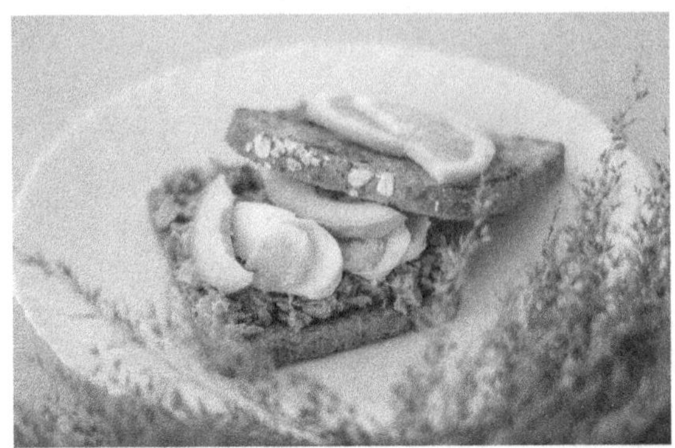

<u>**Whole Wheat Toast with Avocado**</u>

Ingredients:
- 1 slice whole wheat toast
- 1/2 avocado, mashed
- Sprinkle of black pepper

Preparation:
- Spread mashed avocado on whole wheat toast.
- Sprinkle with black pepper.

Nutritional Value:
- Calories: 200
- Protein: 4g
- Fibre: 5g
- Healthy Fats: 10g
- Preparation Time: 5 minutes

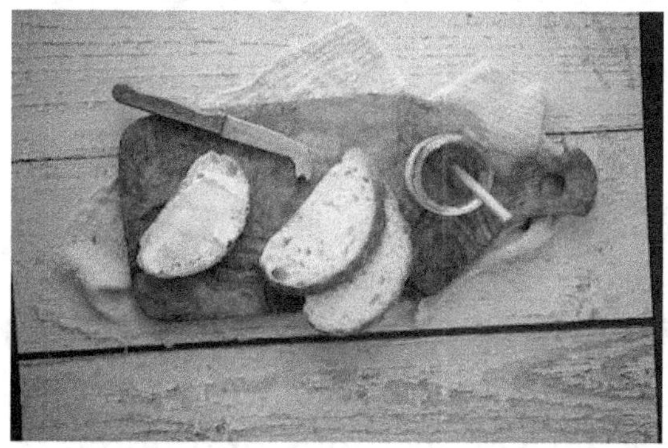

Apple Slices with Almond Butter

Ingredients:
- 1 apple, sliced
- 2 tablespoons almond butter

Preparation:
- Serve apple slices with a side of almond butter for dipping.

Nutritional Value:
- Calories: 220
- Protein: 4g
- Fiber: 6g
- Healthy Fats: 12g
- Preparation Time: 3 minutes

<u>Sliced Bell Peppers with Guacamole</u>

Ingredients:
- Bell pepper slices (various colours)
- Guacamole

Preparation:
- Slice bell peppers into strips.
- Serve with guacamole for dipping.

Nutritional Value:
- Calories: 160
- Protein: 3g
- Fibre: 7g
- Healthy Fats: 10g
- Preparation Time: 5 minutes

These heart-healthy snack recipes are not only satisfying but also packed with nutrients, making them an excellent choice for supporting your cardiovascular health. Adjust portion sizes and ingredients to meet your specific dietary needs and preferences. Enjoy these tasty and nutritious snacks!

CHAPTER 9

<u>Vegetarian Recipes</u>

Vegetarian Recipes for Heart Disease" is your guide to a plant-based culinary journey that prioritises your cardiovascular health without sacrificing flavour. Our collection features an array of mouthwatering dishes that showcase the power of plant-based ingredients in reducing your risk of heart disease. Embrace the benefits of a vegetarian diet and savour the taste of a heart-healthy lifestyle.

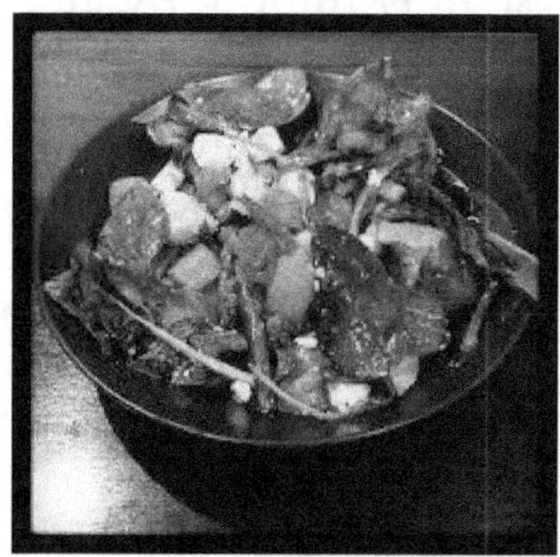

<u>Sweet Potato and Spinach Salad</u>

Ingredients:

- 2 sweet potatoes, peeled and diced
- 2 cups fresh spinach
- 1/4 cup feta cheese, crumbled
- 1/4 cup balsamic vinaigrette
- 1/4 cup walnuts, chopped
- Salt and pepper to taste

Preparation:

- Preheat the oven to 400°F (200°C).
- Toss diced sweet potatoes with olive oil, salt, and pepper.
- Roast sweet potatoes in the preheated oven for about 20-25 minutes until tender and slightly crispy.
- In a large bowl, combine roasted sweet potatoes, fresh spinach, feta cheese, and balsamic vinaigrette.
- Sprinkle with chopped walnuts before serving.

Nutritional Value:

- Calories: 280
- Protein: 6g
- Fiber: 6g

- Healthy Fats: 14g
- Cooking Time: 30 minutes

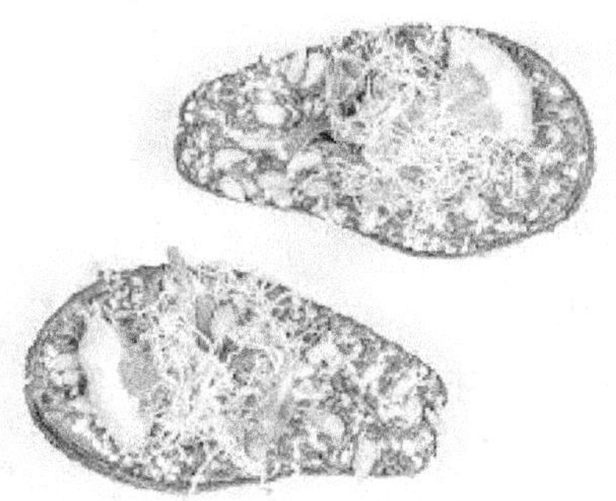

Caprese Stuffed Avocado

Ingredients:
- 2 ripe avocados, halved and pitted
- 1 cup cherry tomatoes, halved
- 1/2 cup fresh mozzarella balls
- 1/4 cup fresh basil, chopped
- 2 tablespoons balsamic glaze
- Salt and pepper to taste

Preparation:
- In a bowl, combine cherry tomatoes, fresh mozzarella balls, and chopped fresh basil.

- Drizzle balsamic glaze over the mixture and season with salt and pepper.
- Fill each avocado half with the Caprese mixture.

Nutritional Value:
- Calories: 250
- Protein: 8g
- Fiber: 8g
- Healthy Fats: 20g
- Cooking Time: 10 minutes

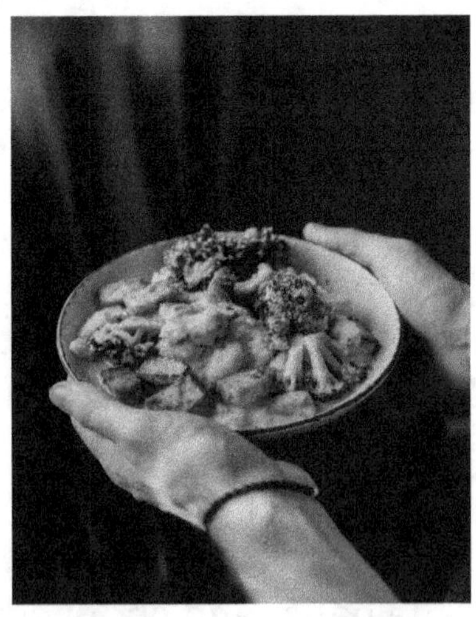

Tofu and Broccoli Stir-Fry

Ingredients:
- 1 block extra-firm tofu, cubed

- 2 cups broccoli florets
- 1 bell pepper, sliced
- 1/4 cup low-sodium teriyaki sauce
- 1 tablespoon sesame oil
- Cooked brown rice for serving

Preparation:
- In a large skillet, heat sesame oil over medium-high heat.
- Add tofu cubes and cook until browned.
- Add broccoli florets and bell pepper slices, sauté until vegetables are tender.
- Pour in low-sodium teriyaki sauce and cook for an additional 2 minutes.
- Serve over cooked brown rice.

Nutritional Value:
- Calories: 320
- Protein: 15g
- Fiber: 8g
- Healthy Fats: 10g
- Cooking Time: 20 minutes

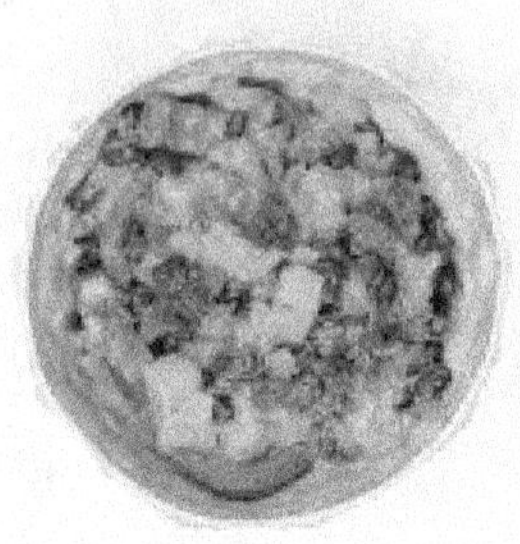

Mushroom and Spinach Quesadilla

Ingredients:

- 2 whole wheat tortillas
- 2 cups fresh spinach
- 1 cup sliced mushrooms
- 1/2 cup shredded mozzarella cheese
- 2 cloves garlic, minced
- 1 tablespoon olive oil
- Salt and pepper to taste

Preparation:

- In a skillet, heat olive oil over medium heat.
- Add minced garlic and sliced mushrooms, sauté until mushrooms are tender.
- Place one whole wheat tortilla in the skillet.

- Sprinkle with shredded mozzarella cheese and top with sautéed mushrooms and fresh spinach.
- Place the second tortilla on top and cook until the cheese is melted and the tortilla is crispy.
- Flip the quesadilla to cook the other side.
- Remove from the skillet and slice into wedges before serving.

Nutritional Value:
- Calories: 280
- Protein: 12g
- Fiber: 6g
- Healthy Fats: 10g
- Cooking Time: 15 minutes

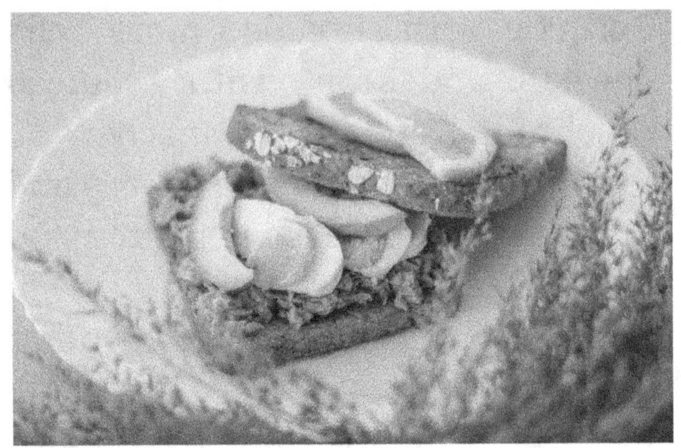

Butternut Squash and Black Bean Chili

Ingredients:

- 2 cups butternut squash, peeled and diced
- 2 cans black beans, rinsed and drained
- 1 can diced tomatoes (no added salt)
- 1 onion, diced
- 2 cloves garlic, minced
- 2 tablespoons chili powder
- 1 tablespoon olive oil
- Salt and pepper to taste

Preparation:

- In a large pot, heat olive oil over medium heat.

- Add diced onions and minced garlic, sauté until softened.
- Stir in chilli powder and cook for 1 minute.
- Add butternut squash, black beans, and diced tomatoes. Simmer for about 20-25 minutes until the squash is tender.
- Season with salt and pepper before serving.

Nutritional Value:
- Calories: 280
- Protein: 10g
- Fiber: 12g
- Healthy Fats: 6g
- Cooking Time: 30 minutes

These heart-healthy vegetarian recipes are not only delicious but also packed with nutrients, making them a fantastic choice for supporting your cardiovascular health. Adjust portion sizes and ingredients to meet your specific dietary needs and preferences. Enjoy these flavorful and nutritious dishes!

CONCLUSION

In this Heart Healthy Disease Cookbook For Beginners 2024, offers a diverse array of delicious and nutritious recipes specifically designed to promote cardiovascular wellness.

We've explored an extensive range of options, from breakfast to dinner, smoothies to snacks, and even delectable vegetarian meals, all with one common goal: to support your heart's health.

Understanding the importance of a heart-healthy diet is the first step in taking charge of your well-being.

By incorporating whole grains, lean proteins, fresh fruits and vegetables, and healthy fats, you're making choices that can significantly reduce the risk of heart disease.

The recipes featured here are not only flavorful but also balanced in terms of essential nutrients, fibre, and healthy fats, providing your body with the sustenance it needs to thrive.

But the journey toward a heart-healthy lifestyle is not solely about food; it's about embracing a holistic approach.

Regular physical activity, stress management, and maintaining a healthy weight all play a crucial role in safeguarding your cardiovascular health.

In closing, we encourage you to embark on this heart-healthy culinary adventure with an open heart and an open mind. These recipes are the building blocks of a happier, healthier life.

By adopting and adapting this diet, you're taking a significant step toward a vibrant future filled with vitality and wellness.

The key to a strong heart is now in your hands, and we believe in your ability to make the choices that will lead to a fulfilling, heart-healthy life. So go ahead, savour the flavours, and cherish the path to a heart that beats with strength and joy.